Unlocking Human Potential: The Art of Motivational Interviewing for Hypnotists

How to Help Clients Talk *Themselves* Into Change

By Christian Skoorsmith, MA, BCH, FNGH

WholeHealth Publishing
Seattle, WA
2023

First Edition, 2023
by WholeHealth Publishing
the imprint of WholeHealth Hypnosis
9451 35th Ave SW, Ste. 200
Seattle, WA 98126
www.WholeHealth.today

2003.9

Contents

About the Author

Christian Skoorsmith is an award-winning mental health professional and elite hypnotist in Seattle, Washington. He is Board Certified by the National Guild of Hypnotists (NGH) and the International Association of Hypnosis Professionals (IAHP). In 2023 he was inducted as a Fellow of the NGH, a distinction fewer than one quarter of 1% of hypnotists achieve. The highest-rated hypnotherapist in the Seattle area, Christian has also been among the 'Top Three Hypnotherapists in Seattle' every year since 2019. In 2023, *The Seattle Times* described him as 'the best alternative therapy in the Pacific Northwest.' In addition to a Masters degree in Religion, he has earned post-graduate certificates in Jungian Psychotherapy, Systemic Sandplay Therapy, and Clinical Supervision.

Known for a dynamic speaking style, cutting edge topics, and evidence-based content, he is a popular presenter on hypnosis across North America, Europe, and Australia, and featured faculty annually at conferences around the United States. Christian is a prolific writer, contributing regularly to two professional hypnosis journals, and the author of several books and training curricula on hypnosis. In 2021 he was given the IAHP 'Science' award for evidence-based work in hypnosis, and the NGH recognized his pioneering work in hypnosis for tinnitus with the 'Hypnotism Research Award' in 2022. In addition to his thriving private practice, he is a husband and father, poet, popular interpreter of Robert Burns poetry, and an OK bagpiper.

Find out more at
www.WholeHealth.today
and www.Skoorsmith.com.

Author Statement

I have found Motivational Interviewing to be entirely congruent with and tremendously beneficial for hypnosis and hypnotherapy. If the working/measurable outcome of hypnosis is evoking motivation and ability to change, MI is a refined and helpful tool in that process. I wanted hypnotists to have access to these insights in a distilled and hypnosis-focused context.

My goal for this book is to provide a resource that a hypnotist could conceivably read in an afternoon, or at least over a weekend, and start applying these principles in their practice the very next day. This slender volume is a summary of a training presentation I prepared for the National Guild of Hypnotists' educational conference in 2023. I deeply appreciate the research, science, and effort that has gone into developing MI, and I based an introductory seminar explicitly on the work of William R. Miller and Stephen Rollnick. I hope readers will be inspired to learn more about MI, and I recommend Miller and Rollnick's sizeable book on the topic as a trove of useful information. As always, there is no substitute for formal training, further reading, and hands-on learning, so I encourage every coach and hypnotist to look more deeply into MI. I intend what follows to be *enticing*, rather than completely satisfying.

My hope in assembling this book is that it offers hypnosis professionals an immediate, concrete application of some elemental tools and perspective that can be of immediate and profound benefit to their work with clients.

I also appreciate Dr. Will Horton and Don Mottin, who each in their own separate ways have for decades provided rich and formative leadership for the professional hypnosis community. Motivational Interviewing seemed especially in line with their contributions – Dr. Will Horton from the perspective of

Neuro-Linguistic Programming, and Don Mottin with his signature emphasis on the clinical importance of establishing quick rapport with clients. I am moved by their willingness to offer their thoughts on this topic here.

The reader will immediately notice the format of this book allowing generous room for marginal notes. This is a *working* reference, a workbook that invites interaction with the reader. There are occasional prompts for significant themes already in the margins to help get you started. I encourage the reader to heavily engage the text – underlining, note-taking, stars, question marks, smiley faces, whatever – to make this condensed material of utmost benefit. Read this book with a pen in hand.

Hypnosis is fundamentally the art of drawing out of a person an openness to suggestion. Of course, all hypnosis is self-hypnosis – a hypnotist cannot make a person do anything they do not want to do – but the mark of a good hypnotist is someone who can help people *want* to do what they 'want to do.' That is where Motivational Interviewing comes in, setting up our clients for their own success from the very start.

I hope this introduction to Motivational Interviewing is useful to you, dear Reader, and am excited to hear how you apply MI to your practice!

CS
August 28, 2023
Seattle, WA

Forward
by Don Mottin

It is rare to have the privilege to be asked to write the forward to such a wonderful training book. Christian Skoorsmith has adapted a technique that will improve the success with almost all clients. Christian has taken a subject that could have been very complicated and hard to use and put it into steps that every hypnotist could integrate into their practice.

Every hypnotist realizes that there are certain steps that should take place in order to have success with their clients. There has been much written on the induction. Hypnotic regression has been studied over the years. The use of Motivational Interviewing is a topic that many hypnotists did not even realize existed. The techniques Christian conveys are wonderful. The techniques follow these three S'! Safe Simple and Short. The safe portion allows the hypnotist to know that the work they do will be safe for the client. If the communication is complicated the client might shut down, so this is where simple comes in. And finally, we have short. Hypnosis is not a technique that was designed to take months to see success.

The approach in this book will stop the client from feeling defensive. Rapport can be reached quickly with Motivational Interviewing. Giving the power back to the client will always increase success.

This book is enjoyable to read, how clients have within them the tools to make the changes that they desire. Every hypnotist will discover totally new techniques to use with every client. Yes, every client will benefit from these techniques.

There were so many wonderful ideas in the book that it was difficult to pick only one. I enjoyed most having the client create positive expectations. Regardless of whether the client has been hypnotized in the past from another hypnotist, or if this session is their first experience, they always have some expectation as to what to expect. With the use of Motivational Interviewing the hypnotist can easily be certain that their expectations will be one of success.

Introduction

by Dr. William D. Horton

In the realms of human consciousness and personal transformation, few individuals have made as profound an impact as Christian Skoorsmith. With a career spanning decades and a reputation that precedes him, Skoorsmith has dedicated his life to unlocking the hidden potential within the human mind. In "Unlocking Human Potential: The Art of Motivational Interviewing for Hypnotists," he hands over a transformative approach that bridges the worlds of hypnosis and coaching, inviting practitioners and their clients to embark on a journey of profound change and empowerment.

Mr. Skoorsmith's work has always transcended the boundaries of traditional hypnosis, blending ancient hypnotic wisdom with modern science. In this book, he shares his years of experience and wisdom, offering a unique perspective on the power of motivational interviewing in the context of hypnotism and coaching. By combining the art of suggestion with empathetic listening and strategic questioning, he is passing along a formula that enables practitioners to ignite motivation, inspire change, and facilitate personal growth in ways never before imagined.

As you turn the pages of this book, you will delve deep into the intricacies of Skoorsmith's approach to motivational interviewing. You will learn how to build genuine rapport with your clients, uncover their innermost desires, and guide them toward achieving their dreams. Whether you are a seasoned hypnotist looking to expand your skill set or a coach seeking a more powerful way to inspire change, the insights within these pages will revolutionize the way you work with clients.

"Motivational Interviewing for Hypnotists" is not just a guide; it is a testament to the limitless potential of the human mind and spirit. Skoorsmith's insights and practical application will empower you to become a catalyst for transformation, helping your clients break free from limiting beliefs and harness their inner strength.

Prepare to embark on a transformative journey with Christian Skoorsmith, as he guides you through the art of motivational interviewing, revealing the keys to unlocking the immense potential that resides within each of us. It is time to awaken the hypnotist and coach within you, and together, we will unleash the boundless possibilities of the human soul.

The only problem I have with this book is that I didn't write it. So don't read this book, devour it, and use the information. It will repay you in ways that will surprise and delight you.

Part I
Orientation & Central Ideas

The time *before* clients close their eyes is perhaps the biggest missed opportunity for hypnotists and mindset coaches. Those moments are usually filled with intake dialog, a more or less canned speech about the nature of hypnosis or the work ahead, or at worst idle chit-chat. The desire to establish close rapport with clients is often so great that newer hypnotists and coaches tiptoe through the 'pre-hypnosis interview' or treat the exchange with kid-gloves, eager to seem approachable and later get to the 'real' work of hypnotizing the client for change. This is entirely the wrong approach to take.

If we wait until we begin our formal induction to start shifting our client's consciousness and disposition toward the change they have identified for themselves, it is almost too late. Our first encounter with our clients' Unconscious is when we are conversing with their Conscious. It is of utmost importance that all our work with clients – in and out of formal hypnosis – is strategically crafted to mobilize our clients' conscious and unconscious resources for change.

Deliberately shaping the 'pre-hypnosis' conversation to help clients convince themselves to change – that they can and will change – is the work of Motivational Interviewing. 'MI' is not a gimmick, a power play, or a technique to trick clients or to manipulate them outside of their conscious awareness. It isn't a simple series of questions one can ask that acts like a 'magic bullet' to knock out resistance. And it doesn't make these conversations with clients *easier* – in fact, MI takes work and energy and focus, and will likely be *harder* for hypnotists and coaches... at least at the beginning. But it is a tool that pays golden dividends, in terms of client motivation for change and openness to suggestion.

Motivational Interviewing is an attitude or an approach to crafting conversation for the explicit purpose of utilizing and moving through ambivalence, in order to help people talk themselves into change, based on their own values and interests. It is about making every word count. MI pays attention to our natural language about change, and thus walks hand-in-hand with much of the training and expertise that hypnotists and coaches work within every day. As hypnotists, we pay close attention to language, we know the power of phrasing to affect (and effect) drive, perspective, and openness. So MI is a natural adjunct to the work many of us are already doing – only focusing those tools on the conversation *outside* of hypnosis and *for* working through dynamics of client ambivalence.

Motivational Interviewing is not a single technique – it is an integrated set of interviewing skills.

Motivational Interviewing as a formal concept was developed by William R. Miller and Stephen Rollnick, starting in the 1980s. Originally, it was crafted to help people struggling with drug addictions work through the compelling and mixed feelings of ambivalence about change. Over the decades since, it has grown in both scope and practice, being applied in almost every discipline, and having been tested and refined through 25,000 peer-reviewed articles and more than 200 randomized trials. It is still a growing body of work, and Miller and Rollnick's signature work on the subject (<u>Motivational Interviewing: Helping People Change</u>, 3rd ed., 2013) itself has gone through major revisions over the years. Miller and Rollnick's book is absolute gold if you are interested in learning more about these techniques and the larger application of MI, and I recommend it heartily.

In psychological orientation, Miller and Rollnick are downstream of Carl Rogers, a people- or client-oriented psychologist, who is himself in some ways downstream of the work of Carl G. Jung. Anyone already familiar with Rogers' thought will see it shine through in MI. However, MI is not the same as Rogers' client-centered 'nondirective' counseling approach. In MI, the work is intentional and strategic, moving toward a particular goal.

As a point of disclosure, I find more personal resonance with Jung, and have taken time in this book to lift up some important themes from that orientation that are not common in the MI literature. I have also tried not to burden the text with too many academic

Carl Rogers

references, but have occasionally included them when it seemed important to or after quotations.

There are many 'styles' of communication. In the parlance of hypnosis there are the historical (and rather dated) terms 'paternal' and 'maternal' to denote a stronger, more directing style and a gentler, almost following tone, respectively. Historically, the commanding and authoritative tone was assumed to be essential for effective hypnosis. Manuals and stories are replete with the hypnotist suddenly yelling 'SLEEP!' at some point in the induction. While it is true that surprise is one way to induce hypnosis and circumvent the 'critical factor' to deliver suggestions directly to the subconscious mind, such overt and theatrical measures have largely fallen out of favor in recent decades.

Perhaps rising out of the invitational style of Carl Rogers or the non-confrontational ethic that rose up in the therapeutic and quasi-therapeutic communities in the US in the 1980s and early 90s, for a time a significantly more gentle, invitational approach gained popularity among many hypnotists. Students and practitioners of Neuro-Linguistic Programming (NLP) will quickly recognize the utility and liabilities present in each of these language patterns, and note the value of using *both* when appropriate.

If one were to imagine a continuum, between a 'directing' style on one extreme and a 'following' style on the other, somewhere in the middle might be conceived as a 'guiding' style. This is the ideal overall orientation of MI: providing guidance to clients without directing them, allowing clients the freedom to *choose* while helping them understand the choice they really want to make. To drive home the idea, Miller and Rollnick list some verbs that might be associated with each style:

Directing	Guiding	Following
Administer	Accompany	Allow
Authorize	Arouse	Attend
Command	Assist	Be Responsive
Lead	Enlighten	Have Faith In
Order	Kindle	Observe
Steer	Offer	Stick To
Take Charge	Show	Take Interest In
Tell	Take Along	Value

You can quickly sense the different 'feel' of each style. While the list might lean toward extremes for the sake of illustration, it is not difficult to imagine tone, phrasing, word choice, and energy that would reflect each 'style.' Motivational Interviewing as much as possible rests in the middle category: arousing and kindling within the client their own understanding, reasoning, and motivation. This is actively participatory for the hypnotist, too! We are not passive witnesses to our clients' growth, but guides familiar with the territory who help prepare and motivate our clients to make the journey themselves. Our role is to summon the resources of the client so they can achieve their goals – sensing within themselves the capacity and capability for meaningful change, and an awareness of their own resilience to see their success even through difficult times of adversity. We do not tell the client where to go, but we also do not simply follow, letting them lead without our assistance. This 'guiding' disposition is essential for helping clients navigate change without dependence on the hypnotist or coach.

In the decades since the mid-20th century, psychology has become increasingly aware of the active role of the clinician's own mind – unconscious biases, reactions, intentions, even reflexes. This issue is sometimes referred to as 'Self-of-Therapist' – as in 'the need to pay attention to it' – or by the older term 'countertransference.' 'Transference' dates back to Freud, who assumed that the therapist acted as an entirely neutral agent, so any impressions, thoughts, misunderstandings, or associations by the client about the therapist were therefore entirely projections of the client's unconscious mind. This 'transference' of unconscious material was of tremendous interest to Freud, who enjoyed a confidence in his own mind and method that often bordered on arrogance.

Jung recognized that the clinician also had their own conscious and unconscious biases and behaviors, and was almost as likely as the patient to project meaning onto the client or their session. To clarify the difference (of orientation, not of essential quality) he termed this *counter*transference. We do not need to dive too deeply into this topic to recognize the phenomenon in ourselves: everyone is, to some extent, always 'projecting' unconscious assumptions and agendas onto others and our interactions. Sometimes it is a source of amusement (like in Shakespeare's comedies *A Comedy of Errors* and *Twelfth Night*), sometimes put to political capital (as in using 'dog whistles,' words or phrases that mean different things to different populations at the same time), and sometimes tragic (when couples pour their own insecurities and assumptions into irreconcilable arguments). As helping coaches and hypnotists, however, it is helpful to keep in mind a simple illustration:

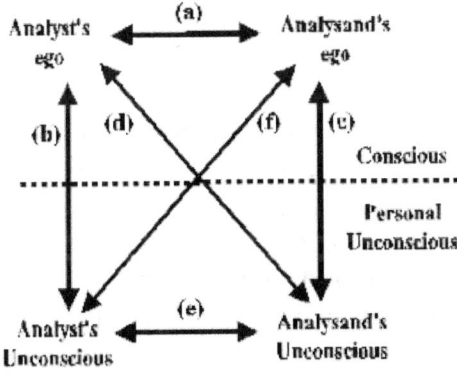

This graphic uses the language of Jungian analysis, but it is easily interpreted into common speech. We have on one obvious level the interaction between the clinician and the client's conscious minds (a) – the overt conversation or speech that is happening. At the same time, of course, the clinician's Unconscious is also active, making assumptions, processing feelings, juggling expectations, and so on (b). This same thing is happening within the client (c); sometimes we are consciously aware of it, but often it is happening outside of conscious awareness. The 'transference' and 'counter-transference' occurs between the clinician's and client's unconscious, interacting with what is being said and done by the other (d & f). One can imagine the startling moment that a clinician became aware of their own deep and undeniable humanity, realizing they too had 'issues' at play in the interaction!

One aspect that was theorized by Jung was the unconscious interaction of the client's and clinician's unconscious minds (e). This has since been confirmed in recent decades with the discovery of 'mirror neurons' which seek out and exchange signals among other people nearby to regulate appropriate emotion, intention, or orientation. This is done out of conscious awareness! We are all constantly networking with each other to establish how we should feel about a given situation or

8

information. Much can be said about this neuro-psychological phenomenon, but the important factor for us is that our client's sense of safety and orientation is in part regulated by *our* unconscious communications, whether or not *we* believe the interaction is safe.

This is why it is of utmost importance that, as hypnotists and coaches, we are constantly regulating ourselves – addressing our own conscious and unconscious issues in healthy ways, orienting ourselves toward positivity and hopefulness, holding an attitude of openness and judgment-free curiosity toward our clients – because we are communicating that to our clients even outside the tone of voice or language patterns we consciously choose. A full treatment of this idea is beyond the scope of this book, but one key facet of this inter-mind-relationship is central to Motivational Interviewing: 'the Righting Reflex.'

'The Righting Reflex' is the desire to 'fix' what seems wrong with people, and set them promptly on a better course. Naturally, this is contingent on one's own perception and belief of what is wrong and needful of 'fixing,' and what is a 'better course.' Typically, this impulse is accompanied by a *directing* style of communication implying 'I know better; do *this*.' This 'reflex' is understandable and natural – even as it is unhelpful and counterproductive. It is also grounded in a profound misunderstanding about the other person.

The Righting Reflex

9

The righting reflex often involves the belief that you must *convince* or *persuade* the other person to do 'the right thing.' It assumes the other person is simply not understanding clearly, or is lacking essential information or important perspective. Therefore, the logic goes, all one needs to do is 'say the right thing.'

Take a smoking cessation client, for instance. Virtually every smoker I have ever worked with already knew far more about the detrimental effects of smoking than I did. Smokers already know the damage they are doing to their lungs, the fact that they stink, that people don't want their kids around them. They already feel the side-glances, the tsk-tsk-tsk sounds people make underneath their breath or the overt disgust they express when passing by a clutch of smokers outside a restaurant. They already know how much money they are spending on cigarettes, and how much the habit is affecting their health insurance rates. There is virtually nothing that I could say that would be 'news' to any smoker. They don't need more information – they don't need 'convincing.' Moreover, if I approached a conversation with them as if all they needed was one more bit of information and then they would easily conclude 'oh, I didn't know that, now I'll quit smoking!' they would dismiss me as arrogant and condescending. And they'd be right!

The righting reflex is a fantasy about my own power to effect change in others – and it is an unhelpful lie. When I respond from this reflex, I take up the 'good' side of the argument, and expect the other to respond: 'Oh, I see now! Thanks! I'll change now.' Reality is much messier.

In contrast to the fantasy of the righting reflex, in reality both 'sides' are already inside the client. In fact, if both sides weren't in the client already, they wouldn't be in our office wanting to make the change! Either they would *not* want to make the change, or they would have already made the change. This is the fundamental nature of ambivalence.

Both sides in client

Ambivalence is the presence of *both* convictions in a person, vying for charge and direction. The nature of ambivalence always lifts up 'the other' position. There is a natural 'yes, but...' phenomenon within ambivalence, always vacillating between the two positions. This quality of ambivalence is important for realizing what we are trying to do with clients and how Motivational Interviewing can help us (and them!).

The normal nature of ambivalence ('yes, but...') takes up the *opposing* position, often unconsciously. The righting reflex actually encourages the listener to unconsciously argue *against* the change. The reality is that, all other things being equal, people implicitly trust their own opinions more than those of others. So, causing someone to verbalize one side of the argument moves the balance of opinion in that direction. (Bem, 1967, 1972)

Miller and Rollnick summarized the problem well: "If you are arguing for change and your client is arguing against it, you've got it exactly backward."

If a client is experiencing ambivalence and we respond out of a 'righting reflex', the client may feel any number of defensive, dismissed, or discouraged feelings: annoyed, not heard, not understood, judged, ashamed, overwhelmed, eager to leave, disengaged, or even oppositional and unwilling to change. In fact, Miller and Rollnick point out that "sometimes in this interaction the person being 'helped' concludes that they *don't* want to make the change!"

If, on the other hand, we were to simply argue *against* the change, hoping our clients would subconsciously take up the argument *for* it, we run the risk of alienating our client and possibly convincing them not to make the change. Doing so would also be just a sneakier version of the 'righting reflex' - assuming that they just need to be argued into a position.

Ambivalence is a sign of strength   In truth, most people who need to make a change in their lives are ambivalent about doing so. They feel the tug of both sides, they are the rope feeling the tension and back-and-forth in the tug-of-war. Most of our clients will be stuck feeling like this undecidedness is a weakness, a personal fault or flaw. Rather than see ambivalence as a *weakness* in our clients, however, we can shift our understanding to recognize even the deepest ambivalence as an ordinary step in the change process. In fact, ambivalence represents being one step closer to change! If our clients weren't at least ambivalent, they would not be seeking our help to change. That is praiseworthy, encouraging, and a show of personal strength, indeed.

Instead of meeting our clients' mixed feelings with the 'righting reflex,' we might turn to the orientation and tools of Motivational Interviewing. In bold contrast to the righting reflex, MI gives no advice at all. Instead, MI asks strategic questions to elicit from the client their own reasoning and foundation for change. For example:

· Why would you want to make this change?
· How might you go about it in order to succeed?
· What are the three best reasons for you to do it?
· How important is it for you to make this change, and why?
· So what do you think you'll do?

We want to cultivate in our clients their own sense of empowerment to make the decision themselves, for their own reasons. We should be attentive to 'change talk' versus 'sustain talk' and keep drawing our clients to expand on and reinforce their own reasons for leaning in the direction of change. The power and importance of this languaging is a common conviction among hypnotists and coaches, since change-talk is one of our most potent tools. With the orientation and techniques of MI, we can be especially consistent with this core value in our work with clients. In a real way, as we pay attention to 'change talk' (as opposed to

13

'sustain talk'), our clients are writing for us the suggestions we should be giving them when in hypnosis!

There is something sticky about ambivalence. There is a kind of comfort in the discomfort of indecision. A decision – one way or the other – requires a commitment, and any commitment that matters costs something. There is a felt sense of this by our clients, which is why they have come to us for help. Our emphasis and continual return to 'change talk' reinforces the truth they already know but find it difficult to face: the only way out of ambivalence is to choose a direction and follow it.

Fortunately, when we meet our clients' ambivalence with this spirit of openness, encouragement, and confidence, they leave the encounter empowered, feeling more hopeful and able to change, even optimistic. When we do MI well, our clients feel understood, heard, listened to, engaged, safe, accepted and respected. But this takes work on our part.

Motivational Interviewing isn't simply a series of rote questions we ask, in order to check off boxes. It is an emotionally and attentively demanding activity of close listening and shaping one's responses. MI is a collaborative conversation style that strengthens a person's own motivation and commitment to change. Understanding how that happens starts with grounding oneself in the organizing spirit of MI.

The Spirit
of Motivational Interviewing

Motivational Interviewing is grounded in a particular attitude or mindset, a spirit from which it springs and which continues to inform it and us as we walk further through conversations with clients. As hypnotists, we are well acquainted with the importance of our own mental and emotional stance when working with clients. This is compounded when we account for the neurological interconnectedness that is especially meaningful in therapeutic and coaching contexts. So it is important to understand the perspective and orientation that undergirds our work with clients, when endeavoring to use the tools of MI.

The 'spirit of MI', as articulated by Miller and Rollnick, fits into the acronym PACE: Partnership, Acceptance, Compassion, and Evocation. We will walk through each of these.

Partnership is the most pronounced Partnership value in the MI model. These conversations are engaged in 'for' and 'with' the client. They are an active collaboration between experts. The hypnotist or coach is an expert in their field, and the client is the undisputed expert on themselves. Partnership is a good watchword for all the values of MI because it takes two participants working together in good faith to achieve a goal. This work is more like dancing than wrestling; we might be 'the lead' but any dancer worth their salt knows that the partner who 'follows' is just as vibrant and engaged a player, and the lead is responsive to their partner as well.

Acceptance of What Client Brings

'Acceptance' is a larger overarching concept that holds several facets. First, in typically Jungian fashion, we accept what the client brings. This is a familiar concept to most hypnotists as well, explicitly lifted up in NLP as 'utilizing' what already is. Our role is to maintain a judgment-free space, recognizing the inherent and unconditional worth of every human being. We maintain an open and curious stance, looking to help the client find every reason they can and will make the change.

Inherent Worth of Client

We extend this cognitive and emotional security for at least two reasons. First, we want to be genuinely attentive to every positive impulse and resource in the client, and we cannot do that from a position of judgment or condescension. Second, as Carl Rogers pointed out, when people experience themselves as unacceptable, they are immobilized. When they experience themselves as being accepted as they are, they are freed to change. This is a truth applicable far beyond hypnosis and coaching, and it is important to internalize so that our whole being is genuinely and deeply affirming the inherent and inestimable worth of our client.

Accurate Empathy

Acceptance isn't only about the client, however. As helping professionals we should maintain an active interest in and effort to

16

understand the client's internal perspective. With accurate empathy we are able to listen without imposing our own perspective. We seek to genuinely understand our client's perspective (experience, view, values, etc.) while at the same time never losing ourselves in it. We seek to appreciate it and also not be absorbed by it, not having to adopt it as our own. Our job is, after all, to help the client achieve something *new* – we have to understand and appreciate where they are coming from, and also be vigilantly prepared to call them into new understanding and empowerment.

Our 'acceptance' of the client is Client Autonomy unconditional, but it is also strategic. We want to support and foster the autonomy and self-direction of the client. Unlike some psychotherapy models, ideally we want to avoid any dependence of the client on us to achieve their goals. (Otherwise, if they are dependent on us, when we are no longer actively present, they have 'lost' the power to effect or sustain the change.) In the beginning, sometimes, it is necessary to allow the client to rest inside our confidence in their ability to change, to relax in our confidence in this work and these techniques. This is one reason why hypnotists and coaches should work to be genuinely convicted of the efficacy of their techniques and practices, so that confidence can be a resource for our clients if they need it. (While also maintaining, of course, a sense of contingency, always seeking to learn more and refine our understanding and skill, even being open to our own professional transformation. Otherwise we become stagnant and unhelpfully rigid.) We can also model autonomy and self-direction implicitly for our clients – not for them to become 'like us' but so they have a healthy and compelling model for their own sense of empowerment, positivity, and flexibility.

Both Carl Rogers and Carl Jung believed that people, when given the essential therapeutic conditions, will naturally grow in a positive direction, that our Unconscious is always working for wholeness and our job is to help establish those conditions and remove blockages preventing that from taking place. This is powerful perspective for hypnotists and coaches, as professionals on the periphery of the healing arts. We do not need to 'heal' our clients – our clients can (and must) heal themselves. We are more like coaches than surgeons, guiding clients to actions and beliefs that help them achieve their goals, but it is still their efforts, their choices, their own power that brings them there. We can point out the way, but the clients get their under their own steam.

Affirmation   Therefore, our disposition is one of perennial affirmation. We seek to acknowledge the client's strengths and efforts, even reframing with them qualities they might have felt bad about or assumed were faults or failures. Understanding ambivalence itself as a positive step toward change, rather than a weakness or shortcoming, is an example of this. Our own struggle with 'the righting reflex' is another example, because on a practical level it is the opposite of affirmation. 'The righting reflex' is searching for what is 'wrong' with people and then telling them how to fix it. We want to build our clients' sense of their own empowerment and resilience, fostering their native confidence that they can achieve and sustain their desired change.

'Compassion' is an often misunderstood concept in our culture. Compassion isn't simply feeling for another person or being 'nice' to them. It isn't always treating them with kid-gloves or 'going easy' on them. Compassion in the helping arts is actively promoting the other's welfare, giving priority to their needs and best interests. We are willing to put our own comfort and insecurities aside to be genuinely present for our clients in the ways they need us to be. We are not task masters lording power over others (feeding some insecure ego need of our own), but we are not apologetic ninnies hesitantly suggesting weak possibilities hoping our clients will approve of us (feeding a different insecure ego need of ours). We confidently help the client discover and reinforce their own resources, motivation, conviction, and commitment.

Compassion requires oneself to pay close attention to one's own inner dialog, inner conflicts and priorities. We must attend to our own voices and parts that might be influencing our work or mindset with the client, possibly interfering with our being fully present for the client. 'Compassion' continues the conversation

19

of counter-transference first approached in the introduction. It is a skill developed with practice, holding oneself with appreciation and care *and* refocusing and being entirely present with the client *on their terms*. As was articulated above, we want to understand the client (as best we can) without losing the 'as if' quality we hold in our coaching role.

Evocation The last quality in the 'PACE' acronym is 'Evocation.' Evocation is different, of course, from 'invocation.' When we invoke something, we bring it into the mental-emotional space or conversation or moment from 'outside.' Evocation summons or draws something from within – something that was implicitly already there.

In a spirit of evocation, we identify and focus on the strengths and resources the client already has. This shifts the typical 'commodity exchange' entirely around. Too many helping or coaching experiences are modeled after sales or marketing strategies. They cultivate a deficit model, focused on some lack in the client that the coach can fix or fulfill. It comes off as: "I have what you need, and I'm going to give it to you."

Strengths- In the spirit of MI, we cultivate the
Focused opposite perspective. We work on the conviction that people already have within them much of what is needed. We are 'strengths-focused.' Our task is not to 'give' clients what they need, but to evoke it, to call it forth. The root of the word 'education' is *e ducare*, drawing out something as if from a well. This is

a concept that goes back at least as far as Plato, who believed we already possess all knowledge of reality and have only 'forgotten' it in this earthly life – so the task of education is to *remind* people of what they already know. This is oftentimes how it actually feels to learn something – when it clicks or makes sense, it is as if we already knew it and just now recalled it clearly.

Remember one of the realities of human psychology referenced in the introduction, that people implicitly trust their own opinions more than those of others. Blaise Pascal wrote: "People are generally better persuaded by the reasons which they have themselves discovered than by those which have come into the mind of others." This might be why Socrates' teaching method was almost entirely him asking questions of his pupils, challenging them to work things out in their own minds. By summoning clients' own resources, convictions, and conclusions, we are not only empowering them to make *this* change, we are setting them up to have a greater sense of control over their lives in general. We are fostering *their* strengths, rather than flexing our own. This is profoundly different than the 'paternal' or 'directing' style of hypnosis or coaching typical of the early twentieth century, and subtly different than the more open-ended permissive approach popular in the late twentieth century.

There is a lovely and compelling image in the *Tao Te Ching*: "You are a midwife, assisting at someone else' birth. Facilitate what is happening, rather than what you think ought to be happening. If you must take the lead, lead so that the mother is helped, yet still free and in charge. When the baby is born, the mother will rightly say 'I did it myself!'"

The 'spirit' of Motivational Interviewing is framed by these four qualities: Partnership, Acceptance, Compassion, and Evocation. Each of those play a part and also represent the whole. They aren't 'steps' or 'phases' in a process. They are infused throughout, forming and informing the work as a whole. These are values that are worth lifting up in virtually every part of our work with clients – in and out of formal hypnosis, before and after the induction. They are especially valuable in shaping the *pre*hypnosis work we do with clients, setting the stage and laying the groundwork for the explicit 'reprogramming' to take place 'in hypnosis' and after the session.

With this 'spirit' in mind, let us turn to practicalities and the 'how' of Motivational Interviewing.

Part II

The Method
of Motivational Interviewing:
Four Parallel Processes

As was mentioned at the beginning, MI began in the context of work with addiction and chemical dependency. Originally, the work was conceived as having two phases: building motivation and consolidating commitment. Readers familiar with 12-Step programs might recognize a similar orientation, though there was no formal relationship between 12-Step and MI. It reflects, rather, a shared conception of the work needed, that was prevalent in addiction treatment at the time.

Through decades of application and development, MI shifted, and is now understood as four overlapping processes. They are not 'phases' or 'steps' in the sense that one must do them in an order, or that one is completed before the next. These are understood as happening simultaneously and repeatedly, mutually informing each other and also deserving their own examination.

Overlapping & Simultaneous

These four parallel processes are: Engaging, Focusing, Evoking, and Planning. We will examine each in turn, but it is important to remember that these are not discreet steps in a timeline, but rather activities we should be utilizing (to varying degrees) at all times. It might seem like a lot to keep in mind – which is why MI is not 'simple' or 'easy to do.' However, I think you will see how these ideas can dramatically affect and improve our pre-hypnosis work with clients.

Engaging

'Engaging' is the process in which both parties establish a trusting and respectful working relationship. Most hypnotists will recognize similar language around the importance of 'rapport,' sometimes expressed as being in 'congruence' with clients. One important aspect is that engagement is mutual, it goes both ways. We are not trying to manipulate our clients into choosing a particular action or committing to a pre-determined belief (manipulation stems from the righting reflex). It is also true that the way we feel can and will affect our connection with the person we are trying to help – a reality that we intuitively feel and that neuroscience has in recent decades found to be grounded in our brains and the biology of relationships.

Rapport & Congruence

Engaging is of obvious benefit. Not only does it facilitate a working alliance between client and clinician, which itself is a predictor of outcome, rapport also leads to the client returning for scheduled sessions as well as experiencing positive accountability from the coach.

It helps to be aware of some potential beliefs or perspectives on our part that can hinder engagement. These are like sandtraps on a golf course – they can slow down or sideline our work if we get caught in them. They might surprise us if we aren't mindful of them in advance. They are best to avoid because getting

Hindrances to Engagement

out of them can take a lot of time and effort away from getting where we want to go.

The Assessment Trap One early trap is 'Assessment.' This is particularly a concern when beginning work with a client. If the 'intake' process is regarded as a prerequisite rather than the beginning of treatment, the client may be alienated from the start. It is important to make the 'intake' process itself be the beginning of forward movement with/in the client. This is partly what we are wanting to do with the tools of MI, of course.

In my own practice, I have a rather extensive intake form – but I have taken great care not to ask any question that doesn't matter. I don't ask for any information that I won't use. As a result, I spend a good portion of the first session walking through the intake form with the client, so they have an opportunity to clarify or comment, and so I can ask questions and begin to understand my client's unique perspective. This is not just rapport-building in the sense of a positive disposition and a sense of trust between us. We actively begin shaping the work and shifting the client's mindset.

Benefits Form In my intake paperwork (which I give them in advance of the first session so they have time at home to fill it out and reflect on it), I have a page dedicated to listing the 'benefits' of the change they want to make. The activity of conceiving of, focusing on, and listing out these benefits starts the process of focusing on a future where they have made the change (maybe even previvifying that experience), it

26

provides incentives for making the change, and it also provides explicit suggestions for reinforcement in hypnosis. Just by filling in the form, we have already started effecting the desired change.

We walk through the benefits together, the client clarifying, commenting and expanding on them as we go. (This provides me more understanding and also more explicit verbiage for suggestions in hypnosis. This is gold from my client – I write it all down.) But there is one phenomenon that is almost always present, and it provides our first explicit learning-moment.

Typically, when people start to identify the reasons they want to make the change, or how their lives will be different and better for having made that change, they focus on what they *don't* want to experience anymore: less stress, won't be so angry, won't yell at my wife, kids won't be scared of me, and so on. After listening to the first such example and affirming their noble desire, I lift up a quality of the subconscious mind. I explain that the subconscious is not good at recognizing 'negatives.' For example, if I asked you to *not* think of a pink elephant, you would likely first think of one and then try to push it out of your mind. If I really didn't want you to think of a pink elephant, I shouldn't even bring it up, and should instead bring up what I *do* want you to have in mind. So, while it is good to know what you *don't* want, I tell my clients, it is really important for us to land on what you *do* want.

How do you *want* to feel when things get stressful at home? How do you *want* to respond when your kids are obstinate? How do you *want* to feel when you are called on to present an idea at work? This subtle shift with clients takes our 'intake process' right into coaching. There is no 'wasted time', no prerequisite or boxes to be checked off before we can start working together. All of our work is important and formative.

This hearkens back to the values of appreciating what the client brings and affirming their innate worth. It also demonstrates the immediate application of the work we will be doing (setting up a positive expectation for our session as a whole); and my enthusiasm and confidence in the work they will do and progress they will experience.

Do not get stuck in the trap of over-formalizing the intake or being officious in an assessment. (One might ask oneself if seeming unnecessarily formal – or casual – is compensating for an unacknowledged insecurity or emotional need on one's own part. If so, do what is necessary to set it aside so you can be present for your client without judgment. If you need to, seek help from a trusted professional yourself.)

The Expert Trap

Related to that is another danger: the expert trap. This is where one assumes the unequivocal position as *the* expert. Remember that this work requires a partnership, and recognizing that the client is the expert on themselves. When we ask questions or make statements that imply "I am in control here," or "I have the answer and I will give it to you," we are disrupting that rapport and sense of trust. The reality is that we do not have the answers for our clients without their collaboration and expertise.

Another folly particularly prone among newer hypnotists and coaches is 'the premature focus trap.' This is when we – even out of an abundance of well-meaning enthusiasm – jump to a conclusion about what the client's issue is and how to solve it. This often results from excitement about a theoretical model into which we filter (or cram) experience into. Additionally, when we try to start solving a problem before we have established a working collaboration, we end up rupturing rapport and trust instead of building it. In reflection, when this happens, we can see that we were trying to direct the conversation to what *we* thought was the problem, instead of starting with the client's concerns. MI is a helpful check to this tendency, reminding us to maintain a stance of curiosity and support, asking many more questions than any amount of offering advice. **The Premature Focus Trap**

Another potential pitfall is common to both clinicians and clients: the blaming trap. This is grounded in the client's or hypnotist's concern or defensiveness about blaming. We all know people who project responsibility or power onto others – sometimes with justification, oftentimes unhelpfully. In the context of our work with clients, however, blaming is only so helpful. Blaming reinforces **The Blaming Trap** the client's 'victim' position and limits their ability to change, to take their destiny in their own hands. It is important to compassionately redirect the conversation away from 'sustain talk' toward 'change talk.' If blame-talk seems a persistent problem, you might try saying something like: "I'm not as interested in looking for who's to blame, as I am interested in what's troubling you, and what you might be able to do about it."

Finally, what might be the sneakiest behavior to disrupt rapport and fruitful collaboration: the 'chat trap.' In our endeavor to connect on a personal level, seem approachable and interested in our clients as unique individuals, or perhaps in an earnest desire to affirm our clients' felt sense of worth, we might spend excessive time in idle banter or small talk. This is a particularly dangerous habit for newer helping professionals, who might lean on informality to 'do the work' because of an insecurity about themselves, their skills or abilities to handle the task, or an avoidance of a difficult or touchy subject. Chit-chat is a real danger, because it is so easy and because it negatively impacts client outcomes. In one treatment study, in fact, higher levels of in-session informal chat predicted lower levels of client motivation for change and retention. (Bamatter, et al., 2010) It has the net opposite effect than likely intended!

To help us stay focused on what mindset and behaviors to maintain toward our clients, to prepare them for the change-work ahead – there are five basic issues to attend to. First is **why is this person coming to see you now?** What do they want? Be sure to ask *and listen.*

A close follow up consideration is your sense of **how important the client's goals may be**. Without allowing our own values and viewpoint to dominate, a fair question to ask is: how significant is the goal? The less significant it is, it might signal a lack of confidence by the client that they can achieve any meaningful change at all. This might indicate to you that more work needs to be done reframing their native abilities and capabilities – either in the pre-hypnosis coaching or in the formal hypnosis session.

William James, educator and pioneer of pragmatism as a philosophy, posed this challenge: if the answer to the question doesn't matter, then the question doesn't matter. In other words, if what we are struggling with makes no difference one way or the other, then what we're struggling with isn't worth the energy or effort – it makes no difference. Of course, 'difference' is relative, but I think the point is still valuable. If our client's goal doesn't make a difference in their life, then we might explore with them why they should focus on that change at all.

Another issue to be sensitive to in endeavoring to engage with your client is **being welcoming**. Related to affirming what your client brings, look for what you can genuinely appreciate and comment positively on – even something simple – and for other ways to make the client feel welcome. Sometimes a smoking cessation client will come in for their second session feeling deflated and disappointed because they still smoked a couple cigarettes since we met. I ask them (again) how much they *used* to smoke and then contrast that with the almost-trivial amount they did smoke. This reframes their behavior in a positive light, as progress toward their goal, and also sets them up to be immeasurably closer to their goal of giving it up entirely. A powerful way to frame this is using percentages – a 400% drop in smoking sounds far more impressive than 'still smoking two cigarettes from having smoked a pack and-a-half a day.'

Especially in initial consultations and intake sessions, it is also good to get a bead on how this person thinks **you might be able to help them**. Conversely, you should provide the client with some sense of what to reasonably expect from you and your work together.

Finally, and this cannot be overstated, we should **offer hope**. The best part of your consultation patter or your intake 'script' should be an explanation of what you do and how it can help. Present an honest picture of the efficacy of your services, so the client can make an informed decision. Frame your description deliberately so it sets them up to have confidence in you and also an awareness of their own role and responsibility, landing on your unequivocal confidence in *their* ability to make the change they are seeking.

The literature of MI offers guidance in OARS crafting communication for effective engagement. One of the most helpful frameworks for guiding conversations can fit into the acronym OARS: ask Open questions, be Affirming, Reflect, and Summarize. Some of these will be familiar to most readers (still worth repeating), while some advice will be new and tremendously useful.

First, ask open questions. Yes/No Open Questions questions or even multiple choice questions are 'closed' questions. They can usually be answered with one word, then the exchange is done. Open questions invite more reflective and expansive answers. For example: "where is that coming from?" and "what does that do for you?" Often, 'open questions' may not even be phrased explicitly as a question: "tell me more about that," or "that's interesting, say more" or "help me understand that a little better." Asking open questions also plays a role in evoking resources in the client to make the change: confidence, resilience, motivation, and vision, among them.

It is important to also be affirming. Be Affirming Recognize and acknowledge what is good. Leaning on our conviction of the client's inherent worth, we are constantly on the lookout for resources or reframes that highlight client abilities, capabilities, adaptations, and positive intentions. Our clients often come to us convinced of (or fearing) their own unworthiness, their own sense of failure or weakness or lack. We have the opportunity to

33

point out all the strengths and nobility in the very elements they've been denigrating themselves for: ambivalence shows progress, reactions demonstrate a desire to defend oneself and assert one's own worth as a human being, even addictions or 'too-much behaviors' are attempts at self-care by providing relief or distraction or a sense of worth (however ultimately self-destructive). We shouldn't be constantly contradicting our clients and make *everything* seem positive (even if it may be) – being sensitive to the most important elements, parts, actions, or regrets, and using those as leverage points to subtly shift their self-talk toward understanding themselves as fundamentally *good*.

Recall Carl Rogers' assertion that when people experience themselves as unacceptable, they are immobilized; but when they are accepted as they are, they experience the freedom to change. From their first encounter with us, clients should feel this sense of safety and acceptance, that we are in their corner, that we can see abundant resources and strength in them and soon so will they.

Reflective Listening In addition to asking open questions and looking for opportunities to affirm our clients' best selves, we can offer open reflections that encourage the client to reflect deeper. Rather than simply asking questions, we might reflect back to the client what we are hearing and perhaps assuming about their thinking. Hearing their own thoughts in different words, or even wanting to clarify or counter the clinician's interpretation, invites the client to go deeper in their own self-reflection. (This is developed further with tools on pages 35 and following.)

At the same time that reflective listening encourages further thought and sharing by the client, it is also a directing tool in that it is by nature selective. We can't reflect every possible aspect of what someone is saying, so we choose what to reflect on, which as a result tends to steer the conversation in a certain direction.

...a directing tool

Summarizing is a further, more strategic form of reflective listening. Summaries are reflections that collect much of what someone has been saying, and offer it back as a sort of package. Summarizing can be used as a way of drawing together a number of otherwise seemingly unconnected threads. It may be an opportunity to link something that was said at an earlier time, or occasionally make a note for the future. Summarizing can also be a way to end a certain train of thought and redirect the conversation in a different theme. It can implicitly wrap up a task or session by pulling together what seems important, or even as a tacit announcement of a shift to something new. In addition to any of the above direction-giving aspects, summarizing is also affirming, as it lets the client know you have been listening carefully and valuing their experience and perspective. Good summaries also have a 'what next?' quality to them, offering the client an opportunity to fill in whatever they feel the clinician has missed.

Summarizing

Note what is missing from OARS: offering advice. Information or offering advice is occasionally appropriate (for example, when a client asks for it), and it is more important to be genuine and present in the conversation than to be frightened of a prohibition on offering one's own perspective. Caution is deserved, however, as we have covered already that unsolicited advice often 'backfires' and works at cross-purposes to the desired effect. When considering offering advice, be sure you have permission from the client. Also, it is of utmost importance that you first understand their perspective and needs, so that instead of simply unloading information one can be judicious about what information or advice and how it is delivered to best contribute to the client's sense of their own empowerment.

OARS lays out the foundational skills for doing MI. As such, we will see them resurfacing in and being informed further by not just the process of 'engaging' but also all the material and processes that follow.

Pregnant Pause

Silence is an important strategy in MI. Jumping in, or filling in silent space is a natural instinct. This draw is especially strong for people who consider themselves an expert in the area under discussion.

Allowing for silent spaces actually gives the client time to digest the information or perspective or question and come up with their own motivation and plans for change. Leaning into the tension of letting a silent space linger for the client to do their internal work, gives them time to reflect and respond more deeply. Of course, clients differ in how much time they need.

A pregnant pause is especially useful after a summary and key question, to increase the likelihood of an intrinsically motivated plan. (Naar & Safren, 2017)

Focusing

Focusing is an ongoing process of seeking and maintaining direction. This isn't simply an issue for attention-deficit clients, there are habitual, cultural, and unconscious factors that often subvert (intentionally or unintentionally) concentration on a significant change. Continuously redirecting a conversation without seeming officious, frustrated, or condescending is a skill, indeed. There is a tension between recognizing that the client-clinician interaction is a conversation, not a transaction, on the one hand, and on the other hand finding one or more specific outcomes that provide direction for the work being undertaken together.

There are a number of issues – on both the hypnotist/coach side as well as the client side – it is helpful to keep in mind, that affect the working pair's ability to maintain a productive and effective focus. Being aware of oneself is a perennial value in any helping profession, but especially in roles such as counseling, coaching, and hypnotherapy where one's unconscious biases can more intimately threaten the emotional and psychological well-being of clients. It is helpful to highlight three issues for the clinician, in particular: tolerating uncertainty, sharing control, and continuously searching for strengths.

Tolerating Uncertainty

Tolerating uncertainty is often an issue for newer hypnotists and coaches, when confidence, proficiency, and insecurity are perhaps unsettled. This delicate skill requires us to resist the righting reflex, and actively support the client's efforts to do this work/change for themselves. This space of unknown outcome is a real risk – what if the client fails? what if they write a bad review? what if they want their money back? what if I am a failure at this career? – and requires the clinician to have an unhurried and uncluttered mind.

There is an irony in this. "If you act like you have only a few minutes, it may take all day; act as if you have all day, and it may take only a few minutes. The difference is in the interviewer's felt sense of urgency." (M. Roberts, 'Slow is Fast', 2001)

One powerful tool is conveyed by the acronym WAIT: 'Why am I talking?' This phrase should be a watchword for all helping professionals. If we are talking to fill the space, to answer our own insecurity, to 'convince' the client, to hurry the process, because we are uncomfortable with silence, because we fear the client may make the wrong choice… if we are speaking for any other reason than to help the client in their own journey, we probably shouldn't be talking. If we are responding to our own issues (conscious or unconscious), we need to set that aside and work on that apart from our time with the client. Part of the value of compassion is, after all, putting our own material aside in order to focus on helping another in the ways they need us to be. The question 'Why am I talking?' helps provide a backstop for our thinking/speaking/acting and

WAIT

reorients us on being entirely present for our client.

The truth is, we cannot always know for certain how things will go – whether our client will succeed, what choice they will make, at what point they will make the change, if ever? Being able to separate our clients' success from our own is an essential act for our ability to be genuinely present for our clients. In order for us to be present for our clients, we must be willing to sit in the unknowing, tolerate the uncertainty, recognizing that this is *their* journey and their success is not up to us (or reflecting anything about us as a person or perhaps even as a professional). 'The righting reflex' is a sneaky thing that creeps up in so many ways in an effort to 'answer' our unconscious needs and desires – but the righting reflex is all about *us*, when our work needs to be about our clients.

Sharing Control

Close on the heels of 'tolerating uncertainty' is sharing control of the work with clients. All hypnosis is self-hypnosis, so we cannot do this *for* clients. Likewise, the work in session (in and out of formal hypnosis) is collaborative. We share 'control' with clients in the confidence that, despite some uncertainty, clarity will emerge.

The analogy of dancing is worth repeating: even if one partner is leading, dancing requires both partners to be fully engaged, responsive, attentive, and to agree on what needs to happen. A good lead-dancer is just as much 'following' as leading! When a couple is really good at dancing together, the positions of lead or follower dissolve, and all that is left is the dance.

An empowering frame of reference for the hypnotist or coach is *not* focusing on the problem, but rather listening for the client's strengths and aspirations for change. Vigilant attention for 'change talk' readies us to find the smallest glimmer: that might be an ember that, if given some air, will start to glow.

Searching for Strengths & Openings for Change

Our clients know more than we do the nature and size of the challenge that confronts them. Oftentimes the perspective they lack is of the resources and capability they also have within them already. Our greatest gift to our clients is the confidence/resilience to see not only *this* challenge through, but also the *next* one they didn't expect to encounter.

To help us reorient toward these strengths and resources, some principles of good practice might be helpful, and begin to lay out a menu of responses, strategies, or directions we might offer clients as we map out possibilities with them.

Principles of Good Practice

Firstly, it is important to keep in our hearts a shared recognition of expertise. As coaches and clinicians, we bring certain expertise to the table – that is why our client has come to us. Our client also brings their expertise, and is the unquestioned expert on themselves.

Shared Expertise

Our most powerful and empowering position in this work with clients is one of curiosity. Naturally, we need to find out what

Curiosity

formation or information the client wants and needs. Our curiosity also goes deeper in wanting to know the underlying *whys*, exploring the *hows*, probing their strengths and wisdom and possibility. It is key to not tell clients what they already know. (Remember the example of my smoking cessation clients: they already know all the reasons they should quit smoking, better and more deeply than I ever could.) We should have clients voice their own reasons for change. The skill of reflective listening (introduced on page 29) can elicit more information and sharing, which can help pinpoint the heart of the concern.

Gently Match Information
When offering information is appropriate, gently match the information to the need. Referring abstractly to 'other people' might allow clients to judge for themselves how this might apply to them. The goal is to empower the *client* to clarify the problem and seek a solution. We might need to set aside our ego or insecurity in order to allow space and invitation for the client to do this. That patience and confidence is the real gift to our clients and the real skill of a helping professional.

Withholding Judgment
Maintaining this safe space for the client to process their own reasons for change requires us also to provisionally withhold judgment about the value of the information presented. The client can tell us what kind of information is helpful. If we pay attention to their lead, we can offer good guidance and information that the client wants, at the right time. This is an opportunity for us to practice

appropriate empathy, seeking to understand where they are while also maintaining an objective stance that allows us to add perspective the client might not be able to see from their vantage point (options, strengths, reality-checks, etc.). A challenge in these conversations is to balance a deliberate guidance of the client with space for the client to identify their own direction and motives. This is the skill of a proficient coach.

As always, we are championing our client's autonomy. Any advice or information or perspective we offer should serve this end. It might be helpful to look at a specific conversational strategy that can be used to focus the work while still being faithful to these principles.

A simple but profound strategy for shaping our contributions to a conversation is this: Elicit – Provide – Elicit. First, *before* providing any information or advice, ask the client's permission. This isn't always an overt question, but should gauge how open the client is to feedback. Offering advice when it is not welcome not only ensures it will not be received well, doing so may rupture rapport and make further conversation more difficult.

Eliciting more information about the client's perspective can help us explore their prior knowledge, and also gauge their interest in whatever information we might have to offer.

When we have discerned that providing information is appropriate, we should consider

Elicit -
Provide -
Elicit

which information to share. Focus on what the person most wants or needs to know. Prioritize the information and start with most-important first. Avoid too much chit-chat or 'softening' which might distract the client, diffuse the clarity of the information, or send the conversation on an unnecessary and unhelpful tangent. Present the information clearly and in manageable doses. This almost certainly means you will not be able to share 'all' your perspective or information. That is ok. It is better to deliver a portion that is received well, than a whole that is rejected and resisted.

Continue to use language that supports the autonomy of the individual. Do not prescribe the client's response – to the information, to the situation, to the difficulty they are facing. Be brief, concise, open-ended, and empowering. Deliberately leave any conclusion open to the client.

After you have shared what you felt was important to share, check back in on the client's understanding, interpretation, or response. Provide space for the client to process and respond to the information. This may require a moment for digestion. One must also be open to the possibility of disagreement, amendment, or even that one misread the situation and the proffered advice was not appropriate or helpful at all. At which point, recognizing the client's expertise in themselves is helpful – we are still learning about them.

This check-in is absolutely necessary and vital – for both the work and the rapport/trust that creates a safe space for the change-work to take place.

'Eliciting' insight, perspective, and information from the client is also a kind of evocation, drawing out of them the material they need to make the change they want to make.

I want to add an element not explicit in Motivational Interviewing. It comes out of research in therapeutic environments, but is helpful in this context. Even if you 'fail' at MI, break rapport, say the wrong thing, ask the wrong kind of question, or cause your client to go in an unhelpful direction, for example, all is not lost. In fact, it might be beneficial in itself, if handled well. Rupture & Repair

For many people, whenever they have experienced a rupture in a relationship (personal, professional, familial, or intimate), it has 'damaged' the relationship, hurt them or the other, or has been a cause for retreat and bad feelings. That doesn't need to be the case.

If we can recognize our 'mistake' (the 'rupture' in the relationship or rapport or even our performance) and allow it to be 'not a big deal,' not stop the beneficial development of the conversation or work, not threaten our own self-esteem or confidence, and instead refocus on the task at hand – this demonstration of resilience and determination can be a model for our clients of how they can themselves experience adversity or 'failure' in their own lives. This allows room for experimentation, and even disagreement, without the threat of disapproval or disintegration.

This is often a new experience for clients who might be people-pleasers or approval-seekers, whose parents or significant caregivers left open wounds after disagreements by never trying to heal them.

Taking the time to address 'ruptures' in the working alliance between coach and client "allows clients to work through interpersonal issues *in vivo*, which in turn may enhance outcome." (Eubanks, *et al.*) In the contrary, simply continuing on with 'techniques as usual' in the context of a rupture may further erode the therapeutic alliance.

While a full treatment of this idea or training in rupture-repair strategies is beyond the scope of this small book, suffice it to say that *not* paying attention to when we might fall out of rapport with clients is even more harmful to the 'therapeutic alliance' than simply falling out of rapport. Research suggests that such ruptures happen often (perhaps in small ways, sometimes larger) in a therapeutic or coaching relationship. On the other hand, acknowledging the break/shortcoming/mistake and addressing it healthfully can actually *help* that felt sense of mutual investment, and benefit clients in building their own sense of resilience, safety, and willingness to be vulnerable.

Field research might even indicate that this 'soft skill' is a stronger indicator for client 'success' and continuing sessions than whatever particular therapeutic technique or orientation is employed by the clinician. (ibid) Unfortunately, there is presently little consensus on what 'rupture-repair' training should concretely look like. The foundational conclusion, however, is clear.

Clinicians, coaches, and hypnotists need to pay attention and be sensitive to tension in the therapeutic alliance, and not shrink from opportunities to repair any potential damage to it. This might be especially intimidating for newer hypnotists or helping professionals, who might disproportionately be people-pleasers or approval-seekers ourselves. Again, the importance of attending to our own issues (conscious and unconscious) is of vital importance in healthy helping of others.

Mobilizing Change Talk – CAT

Language matters. As hypnotists, we know and daily utilize the transformative power of intentional language choice and how it shapes our thinking and feeling, and thereby our actions and perspective. There are examples in our culture (and not just ours!) where speech *does* the very thing it is talking about. When people marry each other, something happens in the act of saying "I do." When someone is sworn into a position in the government, it is effected when they say "I do." The words *make* the change they are describing.

Change talk can sometimes take on this same quality. When we mobilize change talk for our client's goals we should note three different kinds of speech and their respective layers of involvement. The first is **'commitment'** talk, which enlists them in the change they are wanting to make – much like saying "I do" in the examples above.

'Activation' language is approaching the threshold of change, signaling a move from intention to action.

When clients start describing **taking steps**, we know they are engaged. Interestingly, this is the natural playground of hypnosis: moving language into fantasy, from good intention to *pre-living* the experience of achieving change and success. As hypnotists, we are uniquely qualified for and practiced in moving our clients from expressions of desire, to working out plans, to effecting and living out those plans and changes in their lived experience. Using future progression, previvification, and hypnotic hallucination, we can help clients enjoy the benefits of making the change they desire *while* they are making that change, in order to bolster their confidence that they *can* and *will* make the change.

Commitment – Activation – Taking Steps... a nutshell recipe for transformative hypnotic suggestions.

Evoking

Evoking is central to Motivational Interviewing – it is the core of what we are trying to do with clients: helping the client talk themselves into change.

As was said earlier, evocation is different than invocation. When we invoke something – a spirit, an attitude, a memory, a mission, a deity – we are bringing or inviting into the space something from outside that space. When we evoke something, we recognize it as already present in us and are drawing it out, living into it more fully. This is an important cognitive shift when thinking about our clients' native resources. Our clients often come to us thinking we have what they need to succeed. Our task is to explicitly and implicitly cultivate and reinforce their own capacity, capability, and resourced-ness.

Much of the following perspective and advice on how to evoke our clients' readiness for change is itself drawn from the work of Paul Amrhein, a psycholinguist specializing in the language of motivation and commitment.

In setting up preparatory change talk that summons up the desire, resources, confidence, and commitment to change in our clients, we might find the acronym DARN to be helpful in identifying what we're actually aiming to 'draw out.' It stands for Desire, Ability, Reasons, and Need. Clinicians experienced in working with clients toward change may have already employed something like this naturally, developed through their experience. It helps even the most experienced hypnotists and coaches to have these laid out in more detail.

DARN: Desire In order to evoke in the client specific awareness of the dynamics of their desire to change, we should ask them about their desire. This could take the form of simple or direct questions like "How would you like for thing to change?" or "Tell me what you don't like about how things are now?" The latter question focuses on the negative, and so should only be instrumental in helping the client identify the area(s) or behaviors or beliefs they want to change – then followed by positive pursuit of how they want to change them. Another style of question might be more open-ended and visionary, such as "How do you want your life to be different a year from now?" or "What do you wish for in your marriage?"

DARN: Ability A significant move from mere 'identification' of the problem and a desire to change is the evocation of one's ability to make the change. We are summoning this awareness (courage, vision, conviction) in the client for themselves. Questions that might help could look like: "If you really did want to lose weight, how could you do it?" (The conditional 'if you really did want to' softens the question into an even more hypothetical, circumventing the critical factor and any resistance. But I would only recommend using if if there was remaining resistance that needed to be neutralized. If the client's desire has been evoked, *use* it!)

Other questions to evoke the client's belief in their own ability to be successful might be gradually more focusing: "What do you think you might be able to change?" "How confident are you that you could ___ if you made up your mind?" "Of these various options, what seems most possible?"

Sometimes a client genuinely needs to convince themselves of the importance of a change, or some negotiation needs to take place among a client's 'parts' to get everyone on board. At that point, exploring the reasons for changing might be beneficial. You might use 'If... then' questions to chase down consequences (especially long-term ones that might not be as readily apparent). Or invitational questions like "Why would you want to get more exercise?" or "What's the downside of how things are now?" open space for fairly safe reflection by the client. Even direct questions can be appropriate, like "What might be the three best reasons for ___?" (Notice, even in that example, the contingent/hypothetical 'might be' to neutralize resistance to the potential commitment implied by a more concrete answer. This answer allows the client to live into the idea and vision, making it a lure to be chased, instead of it feeling contractually bound and thereby an obligation to be resented.) DARN: Reasons

A final stroke in evoking the importance of the change is to focus on its necessity – why DARN: Need this change needs to happen. There is a danger to these kinds of questions: they might feel like pressure or manipulation. Think of a prototypical used-car salesman who deftly manipulates a potential buyer into purchasing something they really don't want and that does not match the job they need the vehicle for. It feels schmarmy and gross, and we do not want to go back to that person... even to return the car!

When evoking in the client the dynamics of urgency, it is of utmost importance that it is genuinely arising out of the client. Questions like the following should be asked in a tone and intention of curiosity and assistance, without a particular answer in mind or personal investment on the part of clinician.

There are also two aspects to exploring 'need': the importance of the change, and the what needs to change. The first might already be established by the identifying the desire and reasons explored above. If more elucidation would be helpful, simply ask something like "Why do you think this has to change?" "How important is it for you to ___?" There should be no expectation that this answer is exhaustive or final – as the work with your client progresses and deepens, these dynamics may naturally shift, implicitly or explicitly. The important factor here is to start identifying *something* in order to give teeth to the client's conviction and commitment.

Closely following the 'why' is the 'what': "What needs to happen?" "What do you think has to change?" "Complete this sentence: 'I really must ___.'"

When evoking change in our clients, it is also important to be aware of what kinds of questions *not* to ask. What questions *not* to ask Questions that blame, or imply inability, or that focus on a history of failure, are counterproductive. "Why haven't you changed?" "What keeps you from doing this?" "Why do you have to smoke?" "Why aren't you trying harder?" "What's the matter with you?" "What are the three best reasons for you to give up right now?"

As hypnotists, we know that these questions are implicit suggestions, and summon up negativity in the client. These kinds of questions evoke dis-empowerment, discouragement, shame, lack, and failure. Hypnotists know more than virtually any other profession the deep negative programming questions like these can elicit. This kind of 'tough love' is unhelpful and even harmful.

Don't misunderstand me. The questions we have listed here aren't 'easy' or always 'nice.' If our first consideration is treating our client with kid-gloves, we are not doing them or ourselves any favors. We should be encouraging, but also honest and forthright. We do not avoid the difficult questions or topics but at the same time, as Miller and Rollnick put it, distress without hope is no gift.

Be true about the work, but always land on hope.

Planning

Motivating our clients for change, at some point, must include the proverbial tire meeting the road. Planning is a step that moves toward the actual change desired, and can itself be motivating, clarifying, and inspiring. It is also essential for setting our clients up for success.

For hypnotists, this is a natural strategy most clinicians are already using. Planning is important for obvious logistical reasons, but it is also a way to subconsciously previvify, reify, imagine, envision, even live into a 'future' as if it were 'right now.'

One can recognize 'planning' language by its increased 'change talk' and decreased 'sustain talk.' Clients identify steps needed, and might even recognize steps already taken that put them on the journey toward success even now. Planning is envisioning a different future, and builds resolve and resilience.

A simple way to evoke planning is to ask about that envisioned future: How will you know? How will you know you've met your goal? Have a better relationship? At your ideal weight? Have more confidence? Are more energetic and motivated?

This is often the most explicit 'coaching' we do, as we rely on the clients expertise about themselves and draw out of them their ideas, motivation, and intention. We can be even more strategic, however, than simply jumping into 'what are you going to do?'

We want to ask mobilizing questions that evoke activation talk: how ready are you to do that? Are you willing to give that a try? The purpose is not simply 'diagnostic,' to find out 'where they are.' These questions are tools to encourage and help build readiness and commitment. We might press the client in that direction: Are you going to do it? Is that what you intend to do? Mobilizing Questions

Activation & Commitment

Just as in powerful future-pacing or previvification fantasies, details are rich sources of emotion and motivation. We should not be afraid to lead our clients to get more specific: Where would you walk and for how long? (Even what time of day and what days of the week?) How would you get ready? Get Specific

Setting dates, deadlines, and times for fulfillment of actions can be a powerful motivator and measure of accountability. Schedules move fantasies closer to reality: When could you do that? When do you think you'll go? Remember that the purpose of this is to evoke motivation, not overload – and tone can help immensely. Our whole demeanor should communicate our confidence in their ability to succeed, and our excitement about this step toward their goals. Timelines

Mapping out the journey is itself a bold step, especially when moving to the point of detailing what to do, leaning into when to make it happen. Looking at the whole journey can, of course, be overwhelming for some clients. Preparing

55

Losing 100 pounds (or for another client just 15) can seem impossible to envision. One way to help bring the beginning closer and building up the client's resolution is to look closer in the process, rather than further away. Identifying preparations for first/next steps can be a way to make change manageable and model how 'the journey of a thousand miles' is made one step at a time.

For some clients, those first steps might need the most detail or breakdown: What would be a good first step? What would you need to take along?

We want to build our clients expectations of success, and inspire them with being able to enjoy that accomplishment before even having completed it – simply by identifying the next step and their confident ability to achieve it.

Depending on timeline and frequency of sessions, it might be advantageous to set up successive steps: After you've done that (congratulations!), what's next? The next step? What now? What else? Again, however, our purpose with these questions is to empower and encourage, not overwhelm. If we are not building up our clients conviction and capacity with these questions, we should stop this train of thought and return to a tactic that evokes their confidence to take *any* step. The victory is not having a thorough plan for the whole journey, but to motivate the client to start making change. As Dwight D. Eisenhower once said, once the battle begins "plans are useless, but planning is indispensable."

I think Dean Fixen was getting at the same idea with the observation: "In theory there is no difference between theory and practice. In practice, there is."

Opening Thoughts

In their book on Motivational Interviewing, Miller and Rollnick identify three "foci for improving conversation about change inside and outside the consultation." (362) These orienting affirmations seem especially worth lifting up for attention by the professional hypnotist and coach: (1) the importance of the guiding style, (2) recognizing that engagement improves outcomes, and (3) appreciating information exchange as an art.

Importance of Guiding Style At the beginning of this book we looked at the spectrum of leadership styles, with directing and following at each extreme, and guiding in the center. There are times in every relationship when directing is appropriate, as well as following with no particular agenda or intention other than to provide support. "MI is grounded in the middle way, the guiding style, with ample use of following and restrained use of directing." (ibid.)

In brief therapy settings such as hypnosis and coaching, time is often of the essence, and an urgency to 'get the job done and move on' can infuse one's business model and relationship with clients. As we explored earlier, the irony of rushing, direction, and demanding expectations is that they often constrain the individual from making meaningful change. It can also be the refuge of the 'righting reflex', grounded in our own internal insecurities (countertransference) rather than a genuine concern or compassion for our client. It is a tempting place to land, seeing ourselves as *the* authority and unilateral conveyor of knowledge, and that once we have provided our content our job is done.

Grounding ourselves in a communication style and cognitive stance of collaboration and curiosity can be a gift not only to our clients, but to ourselves. As we model this guiding openness, it becomes increasingly internalized in ourselves. While we wrestle with our own 'demons' to make this collaborative and generous position real (linguistically, neurologically, non-verbally), those internal parts of ourselves that might have felt shamed or spoken down to or ordered about, can themselves begin to engage our whole selves with more compassion.

Also, the more we can cultivate this skill with clients, the more facility we will have to use it in other areas of our lives – professionally and personally. Being able to help other people come to their own conclusions and find their own motivation can radically affect our other relationships, management styles, parenting, and how we move in the world. Making people feel appreciated for their perspective and the work that they do, even while considering a change in direction or addressing a vital need, can be a broadly transformative helping activity. "Tolerance of ambiguity and restrained use of directing can be marshalled to good effect outside of clinical consultations." (Miller & Rollnick, p363)

Client engagement is often a barometer of a well-functioning therapeutic relationship (S.D. Miller et al., 2005, 2006). "If the first few moments of a meeting are critical, as many clinicians say they are, then it's not hard to see how engagement" can be critically improved by attending to our first interactions with clients. (Miller & Rollnick, p364) Not only does client engagement discourage drop-out and point toward greater chances of success, for the hypnotist client engagement is of critical importance for many styles of hypnotherapy. If the depth and endurance of a client's change is most affected by one quality on the client's part more than any other, it would be engagement and personal investment in the therapeutic process.

When dealing with clients, especially in a brief therapy context like hypnosis, no communication should be left to chance or idleness. To help us be deliberate in our language and craft our work with excellence, the tools and perspective of MI are reminders of the power in our words and work with clients. Drawing out our clients to lean into their own growth and transformation is the work of those first few moments in consultation and intake. At that point, engagement *is* the therapy.

One of the greatest contributions of MI to how we work with clients might be a greater understanding of how information is exchanged. As hypnotists, we know how information overload can affect (positively and negatively) interactions with clients – not only regarding the critical factor but also in rapport and resistance.

Understanding the professional/clinical relationship as an *exchange* is also a vital shift that reminds us of our own participation in the process, our own need to be open and seek feedback. That is the foundation of the elicit-provide-elicit (ask-tell-ask) model. 'Information' is valuable, but 'formation' is the real goal, and requires and ongoing process of integration, application, and reassessment.

This 'art' of information exchange can affect so many realms of our lives beyond clinical experiences. Avoiding information-dumps while teaching or managing people, eliciting participation from children in the 'lessons' we want them to learn, and motivational speaking, are some examples that quickly come to mind.

"What we learned from MI was that *providing information is a relational matter* and not just a transaction to be traversed." (Miller & Rollnick, p364, my emphasis)

Motivational Interviewing is not a panacea for all client interactions or problems, and is not a simple menu of options from which to choose. It is not a 'protocol' to be walked through, a list of boxes to be checked off. MI is a disposition, a psycho-emotional stance from which to view and direct (even strategically craft) conversations to help clients be on their own best footing for further therapeutic work.

MI doesn't make the consultation or intake process easier, it stands to make it better, more efficient, more powerful. With MI, these vital initial conversations are not a task to get through, they are the beginning of the therapeutic journey itself. The brief coverage of techniques and perspective in this book is, I hope, an invitation to start using these tools in your practice right away, and to further explore them as time and opportunity in our busy schedules allow.

Thank you for your time and earnestness in reading these pages and considering how this information might be utilized in your work with clients, friends, family, and colleagues. Please, do let me know how it goes as you explore applying these ideas in your life!

In the meantime, all the best and every success.

References

Bamatter, W., Carroll, K.M., Anez, L.M., Paris, M.J., Ball, S.A., Nich, C., et al. (2010). Informal discussions in substance abuse treatment sessions with Spanish-speaking clients. *Journal of Substance Abuse Treatment, 39*(4), 353-363.

Bem, D.J. (1967). Self-perception: An alternative interpretation of cognitive dissonance phenomena. *Psychological Review, 74*, 183-200.

Bem, D.J. (1972). Self-perception theory. In L. Berkowitz (Ed.), *Advances in experimental social psychology*(Vol. 6, pp1-62). New York: Academic Press.

Eubanks, C. F., Burckell, L.A., & Goldfried, M.R. (2018) Clinical consensus strategies to repair ruptures in the therapeutic alliance. *Journal of Psychotherapy Integration*, Vol. 28(1), Mar 2018, 60-76.

Miller, S. D., Duncan, B. L., Brown, J., Sorrell, R., & Chalk, M. B. (2006). Using formal client feedback to improve retention and outcome: Making ongoing real-time assessment feasible. *Journal of Brief Therapy, 5*(1), 5-22.

Miller, S. D., Duncan, B.L., Sorrell, R., & Brown, G. S. (2005). The Partner for change outcome management system. *Journal of Clinical Psychology, 61*(2), 199-208.

Miller, W., & Rollnick, S. (2013). *Motivational interviewing: Helping people change.* New York: The Guilford Press.

Naar, S. and Safren, S. (2017). *Motivational Interviewing and CBT: Combining Strategies for Maximum Effectiveness.* New York: The Guilford Press.